50 Sex Positions

The Ultimate Sex Positions Guide:
Spice Up Your Relationship Forever

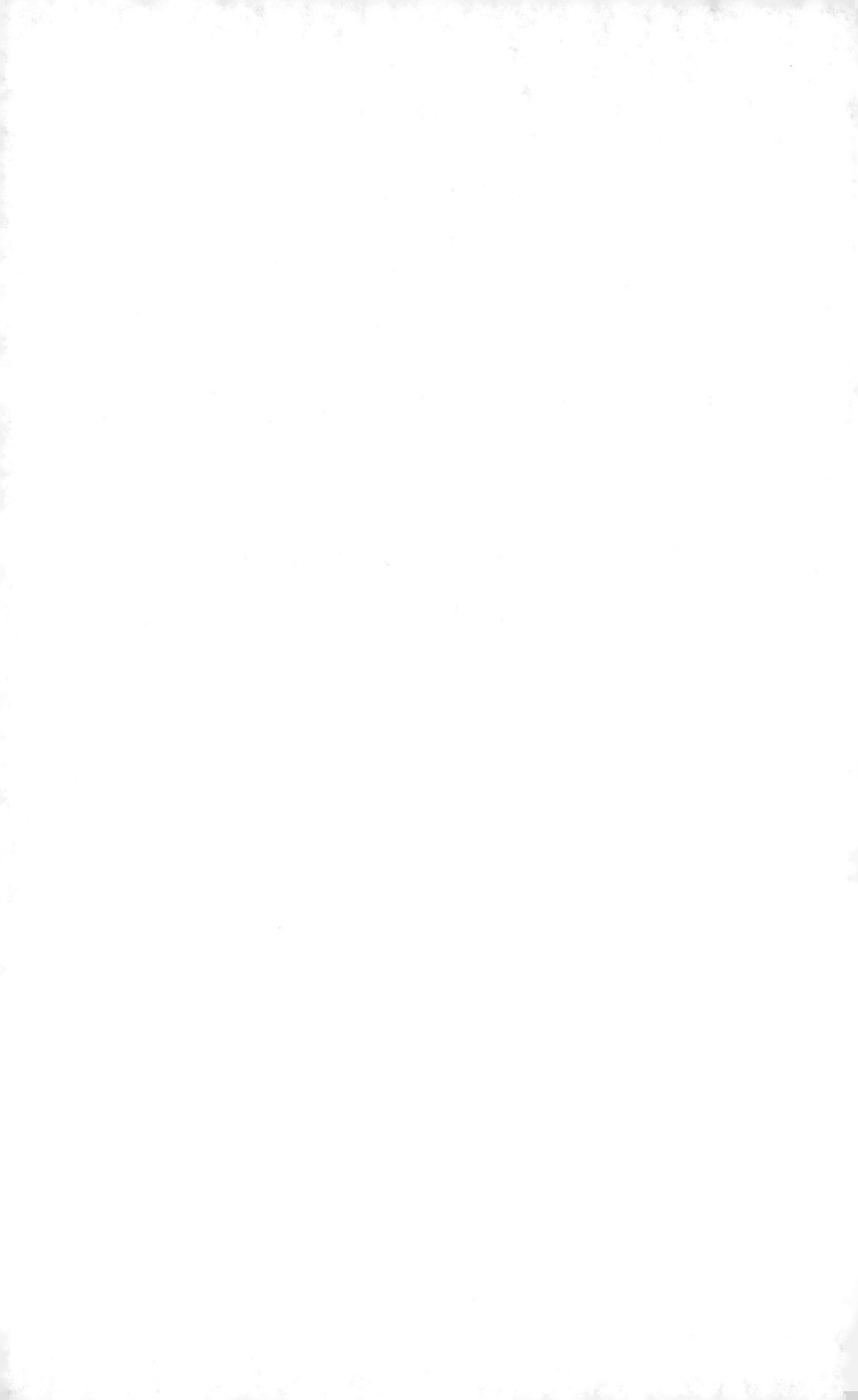

Table of Contents

Introduction

I want to thank you and congratulate you for purchasing the book, 50 Sex Positions. If you're reading this, you must be ready to take your sex life to the next level.

This book contains proven steps and strategies on how to become an expert at keeping things interesting in the bedroom. When you're new to sex, it's hard to know what to do. When you've been married a long time and get into a routine, it can be difficult to keep things interesting. Whichever one applies to you, this book will address both of those scenarios and the best ways to fix them. Not only will you receive some proven tips for spicing up your sex life, but you'll also receive detailed instructions on how to please your partner.

Here's an inescapable fact: you will need to do your research and be willing to experiment if you want to see results from the material discussed in this book. Many people either don't know what to do or are too shy to give something out of the ordinary a try.

If you do not develop your repertoire of sex positions, it's too easy to stagnate with your skills in bed. A satisfying sex life and healthy relationship doesn't just happen. It requires effort and maintenance. To keep a relationship interesting, it's of utmost importance to always be learning and willing to try out different things to find what works and keeps you both fulfilled. This is one of the best ways to become a satisfactory and pleasing partner.

It's time for you to become an amazing performer in sexual situations. With this information I am about to give you, you will be well on your way.

Chapter 1

Tips on How to Spice Things Up
in the Bedroom

If you've ever been married or in a long term partnership, it's possible you're familiar with the phenomenon of the deadened spark. Sadly, many couples know what it's like to notice excitement disappearing from your sex and love life. Even if you do still have sex regularly, chances are, it's not as exciting as it once was. This is completely normal, but contrary to what a lot of people think, it is not inevitable. Why settle for less excitement when you don't have to? There are plenty of ways around this.

You may feel secure in your relationship, regardless of the less exciting sex you now have. You may think that your partnership is stable and that your relationship isn't going anywhere, but even if that's the case, it's no excuse for complacency. Even if you please each other and are the best lovers the other has ever had, there is always room to improve.

If you find yourself in a rut with your sex life, there are some things you may want to give a try to help revive things between you and your loved one. It's important to remember that there are no rights or wrongs when it comes to the subject of love and sex.

Tips for making your love life more exciting:

Try Something New:

When two people have been together for a long time, they tend to get a bit bored and fall into ruts together. It's too easy to slip into a routine and never stop to think about mixing it up or venturing out of the box in the bedroom. Switching up the routine sounds like really easy and simple advice, but it's not always that way. People get into comfortable situations with their partner and are afraid of rocking the boat or saying the wrong thing. Small changes can make all the difference when it comes to this subject.

Speak Up:

In fictional depictions of love and sex, the lead characters always effortlessly roll into the next advanced sex position without talking to each other, asking, or consulting. While this sounds ideal and does happen every so often, it's not realistic to expect this to be the norm. If there is something you or your partner want, you have to speak up about it and ask each other questions.

There is nothing wrong with being more vocal about desires or concerns. This can be as simple as expressing an interest in switching positions. It doesn't have to be a long, fancy speech. Just try to be a bit more vocal about your wants. It's amazing how easy it is to find a common ground once you put your thoughts out there.

Visit a Strip Club with Your Partner:

Many women don't like the idea of going into a strip joint, particularly when they are straight and find no appeal to naked women, but their partners might be totally into it. Some women might be bothered by the idea of witnessing their husband or boyfriend watch other naked females, and if this is the case for you, by all means, don't go this route. For some ladies, on the other hand, this could be a great opportunity to make things more exciting between you and your man. He could find the experience very stimulating and exciting and use this opportunity to go a bit wild on you once you two return home.

Give Your Husband or Boyfriend a Strip Show:

If you're not excited by the idea of watching other women take their clothes off and grind up on you or your man, that's not an issue. You can, instead, take your clothes off and give your man a show. Turn on some of your favorite music, plan out a sexy routine while he is at work, and surprise him when he gets home with your own choreographed lap dance. Some women have even taken lessons! Another benefit of this is the great exercise it gives you, so give it a try, and it's guaranteed your partner will appreciate it.

Role Play:

When you've been with the same person for a long time, it becomes easy to take your spouse or significant other for granted. Role playing can help with this. You can have some fun with pretending like you just met. Make plans to meet up somewhere public and then act like you've never met before and bring each other home.

Another option is dressing up and acting out scenarios, like boss and employee or nurse and patient. Whatever you decide, be creative with it and have some fun. If all of this sounds a bit too "out there" for you, you can always employ these methods mentally for some extra excitement even if you aren't physically acting on them.

Find Out What Each Other's Fantasies Are:

The couples that have real lasting power and can stay happy together year after year are the ones who are willing to open their minds, try new things together, and explore the wonderful world of sex. If you or your partner have sexual fantasies that neither of you have acted on, it's time to give them a try. The exceptions are, of course, if your partner's fantasy makes you uncomfortable for some reason. If it's something that you are intrigued by even the slightest, however, try it out.

Many people keep these ideas to themselves out of fear of coming off as a freak, but find that once they open this part of themselves up to their lover, they're glad they did. Not only does it help you get closer to your loved one, but it deepens trust in each other and confidence in yourself.

Check Out Some Adult Videos to Pre-Game:

It's been said that men are most stimulated by visuals. This is what makes the stripping suggestion a good one, and also the idea of adult videos. Many guys have their own collection of porn or favorites that they watch when their significant other isn't around, so all you have to do is ask him to show it to you so you can enjoy it together.

A lot of guys get self conscious about enjoying porn, so they hide it away so they don't disgust their significant others. Tell him that you are interested in seeing it and that you like these videos too (if it's true, of course). If you're the guy in this situation, try gently approaching the subject to your wife or girlfriend. Even if you've never discussed this subject before, you might be surprised that she watches it too, or has known that you do. Watching things like this can open you up to ideas to try together and take your relationship to the next level.

Make a Sex Tape:

Perhaps you're not big into watching other people's adult videos. If that's the case, why not try making your own? If this idea makes you shudder because of all the celebrity scandal surrounding this subject, get Paris Hilton out of your mind. Making a sex tape can be really exciting and fun. Not only is there the idea of knowing you're being recorded during, but the fact that you can watch it again later to get worked up for a second round.

Obviously, this is an activity you would only reserve for someone you trust completely, or your video could end up online. Even if you have been together a while, but you find that you're still feeling a bit worried, you can always insist that you delete the video immediately after watching it a time or two, or agree to keep your faces out of it.

Give Each Other Sensual Massages:

Depending on your partner and the mood they are in, sometimes just putting your hands on each other is enough to get you going. If that's the case, you must still be in the beginning stages! Whether you're in a new relationship, or a long term committed one, why not warm each other up with a sexy massage? Light some candles, turn the lights down, get in the shower together and then break out the massage oil.

This is the perfect way to get each other in the mood and shower attention on your loved one. Consider throwing a "happy ending" into the mix for your partner, as well. Just make sure you get to the action before either of you gets so relaxed that you fall asleep. Taking turns massaging each other's different parts is a good way to stay awake and ready to get to the sex.

Try Some Sexting:

Does this sound more like something horny teenagers do than two people in a mature relationship? You may want to think again, because this can be great fuel for excitement in a long term relationship. If your partner is at work or out with their friends, it's the perfect chance to send them dirty text messages with details about the sexual acts you'll bestow upon them later. Not only does this make your day more exciting, but it heightens attraction in the relationship. Send your loved one flirty and suggestive text messages and make their day. I guarantee, you won't be able to stop thinking about the time when you meet again.

Start Trying Out Some Dirty Talk:

If you aren't used to doing this in sexual situations, you may be quite shy, but most people love hearing their partner verbally express their thoughts in intimate situations. If you don't know what to say, you can start small with little comments or simple words, like "yes". If this still makes you uncomfortable, try making noises instead. Groan, moan, or whisper.

Noises during sex are one of the best indicators that your partner is doing something right, so don't keep quiet! If you aren't familiar with this avenue of sexual exploration, you may be surprised at how turned on you get when you make noises or express yourself verbally during sex, or how erotic it is to hear your partner speak or make sounds. It's all about experimenting and finding out what works, so give it a chance.

Try Some Phone Sex:

This is for people who are already comfortable with dirty talk, but may make others a bit nervous who are not. If you're confident about using your voice to heighten the mood, set the mood for sex early in the day by calling your partner to have some phone sex. You can get yourself in the mood by drawing yourself a warm bath, lighting candles, and picking up the phone to call your loved one. Get nice and relaxed and into a sensual mood before you call them, that way the vibe comes across when they hear you.

If this is something you have never tried together before, this can be a great surprise for your partner. Call them up and tell them exactly what you want to do to them, use very descriptive words, ask them what they would like you to do and make them answer. Enunciate the words clearly and be "naughty", not too vulgar (unless you two are into that). Pay attention to your partner's reactions to your words and use this to indicate what is exciting to them. Get your partner nice and worked up so that when you finally see each other, you can't wait to hop into bed together. This is a great way to build excitement.

Take Naughty Pictures for Each Other:

If you took the advice in this book about sexting, why stop there? Sexy photos are a great addition to that type of teasing. Your loved one will love to know that you are thinking of them in the middle of the day and see evidence of that through the photos. Something like this can really make a bad day at work seem a bit easier.

Try sending photos to his or her cell phone while you're apart. Or, you can go the old fashioned route and take physical photos to send them in the mail or give as a gift. This shows that you are willing to think outside of the box, do something fun for your partner, and attempt to revive things. If you want to get really advanced with it, you can even take requests for types of photos.

Introduce Toys to the Mix:

If you're a man and your girlfriend or wife has a sex toy collection, this could be a good chance to ask her to show you what it's all about. If you're a woman who has one, your boyfriend or husband may be very interested in seeing your toys. This is a great way to spice things up, instead of withholding that stuff for private pleasure time.

Not only is it erotic to watch or be watched in such personal, intimate situations, but it will also deepen your bond by giving each other a peek into your own worlds. Incorporating sex toys or other props into your intimate life is a great way to get things going. You can even go shopping together to find some. You may feel shy at this prospect, but getting over a slump in your sex life requires looking past that shyness and being brave enough to break out of it.

Take Some Time for Comedy:

This may be a subject you never stopped to think about in regards to sex, but did you know that comedy is great for intimacy? Next time you know you'll be getting frisky with your partner later that night, flip on a funny film. Laughing gets your blood flowing easier, spikes the rate of your heart and heightens the cardiovascular system. These are all elements that improve sexual activity and performance.

If you've been having trouble with stamina, excitement, or just could use a more intense sex life, you may want to consider adding this element to the mix. Start going comedy shopping before partaking in intimacy.

Make Sure You Get Plenty of Exercise:

Are your running shoes collecting dust in the closet? Time to break them out! Similar to the benefits stated above about comedy in relation to sex, exercise improves every aspect of playtime in the bedroom. Not only does it provide aesthetic benefits for your partner, but it improves stamina and helps men to last longer. Studies have shown that sedentary men have more erectile issues, which leads to lowered satisfaction for women. Men who make sure to exercise (even for just a half hour) decrease their risk of erectile dysfunction substantially. You could join a yoga class, take up your morning jog again, start riding bikes together, or get a treadmill. The options are endless, and so are the benefits! Start exercising on your own or with your partner and you won't regret it.

Try Having Sex in Different Places:

It's too easy to get caught in a rut of hopping into bed each time you want to have sex. This does not have to be the case! Try getting naughty in other areas of the house. Rooms you never would have thought to try, or if you live separately, christen each other's homes. If you're the very adventurous type, you might even try having sex outdoors, on the roof, or in one of your offices.

The fact that you could get caught in one of these places adds to the excitement of the sexual act. If all of this sounds a bit too outlandish for you, you could go a simpler route and rent a hotel room for the weekend to get frisky in. Sometimes, a change of scenery is all that's needed to reignite the spark. Don't forget to be vocal and inquisitive and ask your partner where they would like to try things.

Find and Try Out Some New Positions:

This brings me to the crux of this book; new sex positions. Perhaps one of the things you desire most when it comes to sex is trying out new positions. Sometimes, that is all that's missing. Although the suggestions above are good for some people, for others, making this small adjustment will do wonders.

Whether you are new to sex and trying to find the best ways to ease into it, a long term married person who needs some exciting positions, or someone trying to get pregnant, this book will give you some great ideas. There are many positions to try out, and a new one might be just what you need to reconnect with your partner and find that spark again.

Before Trying New Positions, You Should:

Stretch:

Some of these positions require a bit of flexibility to be truly comfortable. That means getting your blood flowing and getting into the habit of stretching out your muscles and limbs before sex. This will take the experience to the next level and enable you to go all out with these adventurous new ideas.

Talk to your partner:

If you and your significant other are in a specific routine and you suddenly try to mix it up without consulting them first, it could get confusing. Asking them casually if they'd like to try something new before getting into a different position is a good idea. Once you find out that they are open to this type of experimentation, you can initiate it without warning next time.

Make sure you feel comfortable:

Some people get uncomfortable at the idea of trying new positions because of self consciousness and how they might look from certain angles. It's important to figure out how best to deal with that type of insecurity. You could start by turning off the lights. Even if a few of these positions end up being awkward, you may just end up laughing together, which is a great aphrodisiac and improves closeness, so you win either way!

So now that we have gone over some ways to bring excitement back into your love life, it's time to get down to some positions to try out. We're going to start with beginner positions for people who are either a new couple or new to sex altogether.

Chapter 2

Beginner Sex Positions

When you're new to sex, or easing into a relationship with a new partner, getting comfortable can take some time. That's why the best idea is just taking it slow and easy, at first. There will always be plenty of time to advance as the relationship progresses. There's no need to rush. Ease into it and give yourselves a chance to loosen up and get to know each other.

Some of these positions are what people would consider "normal", "standard", or even "vanilla" positions. But if you're just starting off in this area, they're the best place to begin. They aren't too advanced or tough on the body, so they shouldn't cause any discomfort or strain, and you will be able to build up some experience and strength before you move on to more adventurous styles of sex.

The great thing about these positions is they can always be adjusted or altered to be more comfortable, exciting, or pleasurable as time goes on. This is a subject you can explore freely with your new partner as soon as you get to know each other more.

Position #1. Missionary

This position has a lame name and an even lamer reputation for being the main position that boring old couples get intimate in, but don't let that turn you off. Sure, it's a classic position and the most "basic" one out there, but there's a reason why it's such a classic! It's really not as bad as some people want to make it seem, and for the person who is new to sex or just getting familiar with a brand new partner, missionary can be the best way to relax and ease into things, while receiving tons of pleasure.

It's also a very intimate and romantic position because it allows for a lot of eye contact. If you're the one on bottom, don't forget to contribute with some hip thrusting, light back scratching, and perhaps a bit of leg wrapping to keep things interesting. This will spice up the routine.

How to do this position: Lie on your back (or have the female lie on her back) with chests together. The best part about this position is the ability to look at each other's faces straight on and also to be able to engage in plenty of kissing, which improves closeness and pleasure. If you're the one on bottom, be sure to participate too instead of just lying there motionless.

How to spice it up: Once you get comfortable with missionary, or with your new partner in general, you can start making small changes to keep the position interesting and exciting for both of you. Don't let it go stale, instead try these tips.

- **Reposition your legs.** When you're on bottom, you can pull your legs in so they're close to your chest. This will change the penetration angle a bit.

- **Pull your legs apart.** When you're in missionary position, you can try spreading your legs further, which will shift the angles of things. If you're the one on top, you can try gentle pushing her legs open wider. Remember to take it slow so you don't injure each other.

- **Squeeze the legs together**. If you're on bottom, this can be similar to a full body hug. Squeeze his body with your thighs to intensify the overall sensations for both of you. If you're the one on top, you can grab her thighs and pull them in toward your body.

- **One foot flat with the other lifted**. Another variation to the most "vanilla" sex position is to lift one leg up in the air to create a different sensation.

Position #2. Pillow Missionary

This is something to try once you've gotten familiar with each other in the missionary position and are ready to take it to the next level. It seems like an insignificant change, but it can alter the sensations quite a bit. Here's how you do it.

How to do this position: When you're ready to start getting down you're your partner, make sure a pillow is placed beneath the hips of the person lying on their back. Then you can enter her or be entered by him as usual. Although this is a simple addition and variation on the position, you may be shocked at how different the feeling is with this new angle. It helps the male's body to press against the woman's clitoris, which is an important factor when it comes to pleasure for the woman. In this position, you can focus more on grinding back and forth than thrusting in and out. It's a good way to switch things up.

How to spice it up: Once you get comfortable in this position, there are ways you can keep it interesting.

- **Special furniture.** Believe it or not, there is furniture on the market designed specifically for this very position. That isn't necessary though for keeping it interesting.

- **Different sized pillows.** To make it fun and exciting after you've gotten used to it, the answer can be as simple as trying thicker pillows or moving from the bed to the couch.

- **Different surfaces**. You can also find areas of the house that offer better leverage. Sometimes a bed can be too soft or hard for certain positions, so try moving to the floor instead. Remember, stay creative and open-minded!

Position #3. Legs Dangling off the Bed

This is another simple variation that can provide a lot of extra stimulation and excitement. Instead of lying in the middle of the bed as people typically do, try moving over to the edge so that your legs can dangle off. Simple things such as having your legs in a new place can provide a whole new twist to sex.

How to do this position: Scoot over to the edge of your bed (or couch) and let your legs dangle off the edge. Allow him to enter you as usual. This won't give you as much control as other positions, but that's also a nice change. If you're the man in this situation, you might be relieved at the leverage this position provides you, and also the level of control you have.

How to spice it up: So having your legs dangling off the bed sounds interesting, but how do you keep it that way? Let's look at some ways to mix it up and keep it exciting.

- **Try adding a pillow.** If your bed isn't the right height for this to work, you can try adding a pillow beneath the hips of the person on bottom. Sometimes, that's all that's needed for the perfect height and level of penetration.

- **Have the male kneel by the bed.** If you are working with a bed that lies very close to the floor, a kneeling position might work better. From here, the man can hold each leg in his arms for better intensity and leverage. If the woman is flexible, she can try resting her ankles on his shoulders for a super intense angle. Be sure to take this slow since the deepness is much more intense this way.

Position #4. Female on Top

This is one we're all somewhat familiar with, even in a purely conceptual way. Any variation of this position is fun when you're new to sex because it offers a lot of control to both parties. Some people, especially those new to sex, may be intimidated by this position and have no idea what to do, but that's okay. Sex is a very instinctual thing. If you're a girl new to sex, this can be great because you set your own rhythm and pace. If you're shy, you can always turn the lights off. This position is great because it works anywhere, and if you're wearing a skirt, it's one of the quickest you can get into, often without even removing any clothes!

How to do this position: If you're the guy, just lie back and enjoy. If you're the female, ask him to lie back, and crawl onto his body, straddling it with your legs. Gently take his penis into your cupped hand and lower yourself onto it. If you are not sufficiently lubricated, it's a good idea to use a lubricant, since this position isn't very nice without the proper level of wetness.

How to spice it up: This isn't a singular position, and there are endless ways to keep it fun and different. If you're the one on top, you can have lots of fun playing around with the speed and intensity of the thrusts.

- **Circular motions.** You can make a grinding, circular motion with your hips. Try alternating from small to large circles, and vice versa.

- **Bouncing up and down.** You can move up and down, either sitting straight up, or leaning forward. Either of these will offer a different angle and level of penetration. You can also alternate between the two.

- **Moving back and forth.** Instead of bouncing up and down or grinding in circles, you can try moving your hips back and forth. This provides amazing clitoral stimulation.

- **Ask what feels best.** Whether you're the one on top or bottom, asking what feels best is a good idea. If you're the girl on top, you can ask the guy to guide your hips in the motion that feels best for him so you can mimic it. If you're the guy, you can encourage her to show you what is ideal for her.

Position #5. In a Chair

This one is great because there's a certain level of spontaneity involved. Even if it's planned out, the fact that it's in a non-typical place adds a level of excitement to the act.

How to do this position: For this position, you need to use the right type of chair. Ideally, it's a short one that doesn't have wheels attached. Armrests can also get in the way for this position, so try to find one without them so you can move freely. Now sit down in a chair or have your man sit down in a chair, slowly lower yourself onto him or encourage her to lower herself onto you.

Again, it's important to be primed for this position, and if you aren't, use some lube or start out with a different position. Keep both feet (or her feet) planted on the ground for extra leverage. She can also hold onto him or the chair for extra support. This arrangement will make the motions easy and effortless.

How to spice it up: Having sex in a chair sounds pretty straightforward, but there are ways to get the optimal experience every time. Some of those suggestions are

- **Turning around.** If the chair is big enough to support you both without the concern of falling off, this is a great idea.

This provides him with a nicer view and makes the overall experience more naughty and exciting.

- **Leaning back.** The female on top can lean back while in the chair sex position. This gives her the chance to play with her clitoris and gives the male a nice view at her entire body and her pleasuring herself.

- **Wearing sexy outfits.** This is the optimal situation to act out a sexy fantasy, particularly in one of your work places. Putting on the right attire can add to the excitement and fantasy even more.

Position #6. **Against the Table**

This is a fun and active position to engage in with your significant other. It's more spontaneous and exciting than the typical scenario of having sex in a bed. While I mention here that it's sex against a table, you can be versatile and use different surfaces as well. If you find something of the right height, this won't be a difficult or uncomfortable position at all.

How to do this position: This is a great position for spontaneous play with your partner. You don't have to plan things out obsessively or be ready to go ahead of time, you can just grab each other and get down to business. This is pretty self-explanatory. If you're the guy, grab your girl and place her on the edge of the table and have at it. If you're the girl, you can take charge, but the table needs to be the right height.

How to spice it up: Some variations of this position are possible to make it even more fun and exciting. Don't get stuck only using one table in one area. Make sure you're branching out to keep it interesting for you and your partner.

- **Initiate this position at work.** If you go to meet your lover while they're at the office, this could be a great chance to lock the door behind you and initiate some action. It makes it even more risky and exciting when you know you might get caught!

- **Introduce some role playing action.** This is the perfect opportunity to have a role play scenario where you and your partner can pretend that you just met. This could involve playing out a scenario where you are colleagues, or just met in a business meeting.

Position #7. **Reverse Cowgirl**

This is a simple variation of the girl on top position. The girl just faces the other direction. Instead of the guy getting a full on look at the woman's front side, he gets to stare at her back and rear, which many men will love. A lot of variations are available for this particular position, which you can ease into as you get to know your partner better and get more comfortable. You will find that the more times you try it, the more naturally the variations will unfold.

How to do this position: It's similar to when you have the girl on top or when you climb on top of your man, but you face the other way. The male is lying back down on the bed (or other surface) and you face his feet, and lower yourself onto him. The angle of penetration is a bit different than the typical girl on top position, so adjust accordingly and find what feels comfortable for you.

How to spice it up: You aren't stuck with just one way of doing reverse cowgirl. Sure, you climb on top with your backside facing the guy, but what next? Let's look at some of the options you have for mixing it up and keeping it intriguing.

- **Move up and down.** You have a couple of options here for reverse cowgirl. You can do the typical motion of moving up and down on his penis, which provides a detailed view for him. This is great, especially if you're with a well-endowed guy, because you can control how much goes up inside.

- **Move back and forth.** This is better for deeper and more intense penetration. You want to make sure you're prepared for this motion, with plenty of natural or added lubrication. You also need to be sure that you and your partner are sufficiently warmed up since this motion goes very deep.

- **Lean back toward him.** As you're on top of the guy, you can lean your body backward, which helps you feel closer to his body for intimacy and also gives you the opportunity to play with your own clitoris. If you're the guy in this situation you can reach up and give her a back massage or place your hands on her hips.

Position #8. Up Against the Wall

This one is great because although it's basic, it's outside of the norm and more exciting than your typical missionary position. It's convenient because you don't need any added implements, just an adventurous spirit and you're ready to go.

How to do this position: This one takes a bit of stamina if you're the one thrusting. This is great for spontaneous intimate moments, and can be done nearly anywhere (depending on how adventurous you are!) Simply grab your partner and get them up against a wall and go to town. It works best if the woman is wearing a skirt.

How to spice it up: There a few ways you can make this classic more interesting of a position in addition to being spontaneous about where you choose to do it.

- **Hold her up against the wall.** This one will take some strong arms, so it's worth getting them in shape. Almost every woman will appreciate being lifted up by you and being made to feel light as a feather.

- **Have her turn around.** This is a quick and easy way to mix up this position. The wall will give her something to hold onto which gives her leverage for more movement or the option for holding herself up while you do most of the movements. In this position, the male will be the one dominating which can be enjoyable for both parties.

Position #9. 69

This isn't a typical sex position that involves penetration, but it's a great warm up and one of the most well known and basic sex acts you can partake in. The idea with this position is giving and receiving pleasure simultaneously. It's very exciting and also helps you feel connected with your partner.

How to do this position: The simplest way to get into the 69 position is both lying on your sides on a bed or other flat and comfortable surface (such as a couch). Then, you give each other oral sex at the same time while doing an equally amount of movements.

Ways to spice it up: There are a few different ways this position can go besides the typical simple way of both lying on your sides. You may find that it's difficult to focus completely on performing this act while it's being done to you, but the challenge makes it fun. To make it more interesting, you can do any of these things.

- **Have the girl on top.** The man will lie flat on his back as the female climbs on top and straddles his face while leaning forward and giving him oral sex. It's ideal to have compatible heights for this.

- **Have the guy on top.** Another option is having the female be the one lying back with the guy doing most of the motion, lowering himself into her mouth as he tends to her down below.

- **Pay attention to each other's rhythms.** You can keep this interesting by paying attention to your partner's breathing and noises and adjust your techniques and pace accordingly. You can even get into a specific, matching rhythm.

Position #10. Standing Up From Behind

This one is an interesting challenge because unlike the wall position, you don't have something solid to hold onto. This one is a great workout for both parties and builds stamina, which is necessary for a great sex relationship. Newbies would do well to add this to their routine to build stamina.

How to do this position: The female will have to make sure she is arching her back sufficiently and enabling him to reach her and may find it easier to bend over with her hands resting on her thighs and supporting her weight. If she finds it easier, she can support her weight using her arms against something like a chair or couch.

How to spice it up: The appeal of this position is how spontaneous it is. It doesn't feel as planned out and predictable as just another evening in bed. To make it even more thrilling, you can do any of these things.

- **Have the guy hold still and do most of the work.** Typically, the man would be the one doing the thrusting in this scenario, and the female would have to focus on her balance. She can, however, ask him to hold still as she does the thrusting motions.

- **Keep your clothes on.** You might be wondering how on earth this could make this position sexier, but getting naughty while you're fully clothed makes it feel more spontaneous and fun. Initiating this position when your partner least expects it is best.

Chapter 3

The Best Sex Positions for Female Orgasm

Most women cannot reach climax from penetration alone, and need special attention and stimulation directed at their clitoris specifically. However, it is possible for some to orgasm from penetration if you do it the right way. The positions that offer the highest probability of getting her off are the ones that put direct stimulation in her most sensitive area. Let's take a look at what those positions are.

Position #11. Girl on Top, Chests Together

In the typical girl on top position, there is only minimal contact with her clitoris, meaning that some sensitive girls could get off this way. There is, however, a variation to this position that will make it more likely.

How to do this position: Start out in the usual position where the girl is the one on top straddling him. Once you start having sex, the female can lean forward with your chests together. If you are very flexible, you may be able to get them low enough to touch. Many women appreciate this position because they may be subconscious about being fully exposed when they are sitting upright, and this offers more intimacy and less of a concern for how she looks.

How to spice it up: This position is better than the typical girl on top scenario because you are closer together, which is necessary for her orgasm. For a lot of women, sex is about emotional closeness, so having faces close together is optimal for that factor.

- **Make a lot of eye contact.** Since she is leaning forward, it presents a better opportunity to get face to face and make some nice eye contact while you're having sex. This can be a very deep feeling and connect you with the person you're sharing this experience with.

- **Make sure there's a lot of kissing.** Kissing is important to many women when it comes to reaching orgasm. In fact, it's necessary for some of them, so don't neglect this aspect of things, and take the opportunity this position presents for easy access to her lips.

- **Have her old still and do the motions yourself.** Although the woman is on top in this position, it's also possible for the man to be the one who exerts control by having her hold still and doing the thrusting himself. For some females, this may be more stimulating and contribute to a great climax.

Position#12. Crisscross

This is another position that offers a great opportunity for plenty of clitoral stimulation. Instead of the man's pubic bone being the source of the friction and thus the orgasm, it offers an opportunity for either the woman or the man to reach down and rub the clit, which is what it takes for many women to climax.

This is a great and versatile position because it gives both parties an option for how much control they want.

How to do this position: Both partners heed to by lying down, with the female on her back and the male lying on his side with his arm supporting his body. The woman will then drape her legs over his groin. Envision a giant X shape. Both partners can move equally or one or the other can take control.

How to spice it up: This is a perfect opportunity for clitoral stimulation using the hands. For many females, this is the easiest way to get off, and most sex positions make this difficult or impossible. This can be done by having the male do the thrusting as she lies back, relaxes, and plays with herself or guides his hands to her clitoris.

Position #13. The Coital Alignment Technique

Many people consider this sex position the greatest in the world for both parties involved. It's an old technique that people have been using to reach simultaneous climax for a long time. Let's look at the mechanics of this position so you can learn to do it.

How to do this position: Begin in the typical missionary style, with the woman lying on her back and the man resting his weight upon her, instead of resting on his own arms. He will now move forward so his pubic bone (the base of his penis) is right up against her clitoris.

How to spice it up: To get the best contact and orgasms possible, the female can't just lie there. Here is how to make sure both parties stay involved.

- **Wrap your legs around him.** This allows for your bodies to be even closer together and for him to reach deeper inside of you. Many men enjoy the embraced feeling this gives him.

- **Rock back and forth together.** The best way to get into a great rhythm is to rock together instead of one or the other doing most of the motion. It can be fun to have your partner do most of the physical activity, but staying in a specific aligned rhythm together creates a better, harmonious sexual connection.

Position #14. Ankles Up

There aren't many positions that allow for full on penetration, including the typical missionary style or some of the standing positions mentioned earlier. That's why this one is so great.

How to do this position: Enjoy the deeper contact this position allows by adjusting the positioning of her legs. She must be a bit flexible for this to be possible, but if she's limber enough, simply hold her ankles up near your shoulders on either side of your neck.

How to spice it up: Depending on how short or tall she is, there are a lot of variations you can do with this position.

- **Hold her in the air.** This would work particularly well with a taller guy and a shorter woman. As you have her ankles over your shoulders, support her weight by holding her hips.

- **Lean forward.** Again, this will only be appreciated by a limber lady, but it's possible to get even deeper into her and reach her G spot by leaning forward so that her body is in a somewhat folded shape. This also allows the opportunity to be eye to eye and to do some kissing.

- **Put her feet on your chest.** A variation of this specific position is having her bend her knees and put the bottoms of her feet against your chest. This may be more comfortable than keeping the legs straight, but doesn't sacrifice any of the deepness that will be so nice for you both.

Position #15. Kneeling

This is a position where both partners are kneeling on the bed or other surface. The reason it's great for the female orgasm is the level of exposure of the clitoris, which means that she can either service herself or he can reach down and do it for her. The positioning makes it easy to reach.

How to do this position: The woman must face away from the man as he kneels behind her to enter from the back. Balance here is important, so this is a good opportunity to take it slow so neither of you fall off the bed.

How to spice it up: This allows for a lot of experimenting due to how free both partners' bodies and hands are. To make this even more arousing, you can do any or all of the following suggestions.

- **Fondle her chest while kissing her neck.** Since this section is about the female attaining an orgasm, you should remember to pay attention to her entire body and to shower it with affection. This position is a great opportunity for doing that.

- **Try it on the bed against the wall.** The wall can provide a great source of leverage for her to support herself up against, giving him more freedom to thrust deeper without knocking her over. The bed also provides a comfortable surface for the knees of both people involved.

- **Try it on the floor.** Some couples may find that it's easier to balance in this position if they get onto the floor and she holds herself up with her hands against a wall. Be warned that this won't be comfortable with a pillow or some other kind of pad underneath the knees, if you're using a hardwood floor.

Position #16. Cowgirl with Bent Legs

We're all familiar with the typical position where the woman kneels and straddles the guy as he's flat on his back, but this variation takes that classic to a different level. Although it's only a small change, it changes the entire dynamic.

How to do this position: The woman gets into the typical girl on top position, but instead of keeping your legs flat, you will bend them to support her butt with your upper legs. This puts less stress on her body and legs and allows her to be in control.

How to spice it up: He can take this opportunity to use his hands to explore her entire body while she focuses on setting the pace and delaying his orgasm if she wants to, so she can reach hers first.

Position #17. The Bridge

This is similar to a yoga position of the same name. For this position, you will start out in the familiar missionary arrangement and then make some small changes for the optimum experience.

How to do this position: Begin with the male on top and the female flat on her back and her feet flat. Now the male will sit up so that he is on his knees before her. After this, she will arch her back so that her butt is up off the bed and her pelvis is roughly equal with yours. By positioning her body to meet the height necessary to reach your penis, the perfect position can be created that allows for the most penetration.

How to spice up this position: There are a couple of ways to keep this one interesting, and tips to keep you both from straining yourselves and having to stop mid-sex.

- **Introduce some pillow into the mix.** Holding her butt up like that can get tiring depending on how long she holds that position. Placing pillows beneath her back will help take some strain off of her thighs.

- **Support her weight with your arms.** This is a great opportunity for him to receive a bit of a workout during sex. As she holds her butt up and meets his pelvis with her vagina, he can wrap her arms around her at the hips and hold her up while he does the thrusting.

Position #18. Belly Down

This one is similar to missionary, but instead of facing you, she is turned the other way. This is an easy position to effortlessly transition into from doggy style or the position where you are both kneeling on the bed with her in front of you, because all you have to do is lean forward, place your weight on her body and press her flat. This position allows for very deep penetration so make sure you start out slow and ensure that she is comfortable.

How to do this position: Have her lie flat on her stomach as you hover over her body. This is a great opportunity to give her some sensual massage to warm her up for what is next. Her legs will be flat against the bed in a straight position and she can raise her butt slightly to make your entry easier. Slide in slowly, remembering that this position may not be as easy to get into as missionary. Some lubricant may be a good idea. Although this is a rear entry position, it also feels very close and intimate, since she can feel his arms around her upper body.

How to spice it up: This position keeps both your bodies close together but allows you both free movement with your hands, which allows for some interesting variations.

- **Massage her body during sex.** This position frees up your hands or at least one of them to wander freely and caress her body. There are many different areas you can reach including the neck and shoulders, her arms, and sides. You will also be in a great position for kissing her around the shoulders or even the cheek.

- **Use a pillow.** This is another position where a pillow can be a great addition, because it adjusts the angle and intensity of penetration. If the man is quite endowed, this addition is probably unnecessary and may even cause a bit of discomfort, but if you and your partner are comfortable together, adding a pillow can add a welcomed twist to the situation.

- **Pay attention to her clitoris or encourage her to.** This is one of the greatest positions for servicing her clitoris. The arrangement of this one makes it easy for her to reach down herself or for him to take over and do the work. This will bring her to an intense orgasm if the motion is consistent.

Position #19. The Bent Waist Position

This one is similar to the classic rear-entry positions but different in that it allows him better control of his body and the momentum of his movements. Since he is standing up, he can get optimal leverage and also better stamina since the entire body is engaged. This arrangement allows her to completely relax, which is optimal for reaching her climax, and also makes her feel dominated which many women crave to get off.

How to do this position: This one is great for manual clitoral stimulation, and involves the man standing near the edge of the bed while she is lying face down with her butt in the air. He enters her as he typically would in doggy style but instead of her having her weight supported on her arms, she's resting on her upper body. This makes it so that her face is buried in the pillow or bed which can feel very erotic and like surrendering to her partner.

How to spice it up: There are a few variations you can apply to this position to keep it exciting and thrilling.

- **Hold her arms down at the waist.** If she enjoys the feeling of being dominated, you could add in this twist. Gently grab her arms and hold her by the hands so that her hands are at her hips with yours on top of them.

- **Provide her with clitoral stimulation.** This one is a great opportunity to play attention to her clitoris, which will be exposed and in a great position for you to reach it.

Position #20. Classic Missionary Position with a Twist

This is similar to the familiar beginner position of missionary, but just a little bit different. This position is easy to transition into from missionary which is great for taking little breaks between sex and also for mixing up the routine to keep it interesting. Since variation is key in an interesting sex session, it's best to start adding this one into your routine.

How to do this position: Each partner should grasp each other and roll over onto their sides from missionary position, supporting their bodies with their arms. You can also adjust the position of your legs to find the right amount of leverage. Making sure your legs are entwined will help you stay balanced instead of feeling lopsided or toppling over.

How to spice it up: There is a lot of room for variation with this position since your bodies are both facing each other with room for movement and entwined together. Both of your hands should be free which leaves a lot of room for stimulating each other's body's with your palms and fingers.

- **Move very slowly.** It can be tempting to get lost in the heat of the moment and pump away, but sometimes it's nice to draw things out and relax a bit. This makes the entire sexual session more intense and satisfying for both partners, and since females usually need longer to reach orgasm, it gives you time to build up to hers. Moving slowly can be the best way to add tension and desire to the mis.

Chapter 4

Sex Positions for Burning the Most Calories

Sex is one of the healthiest activities you can partake in, both for your body and mind. We all know that it provides great exercise, but what if we knew exactly which moves to perform to work out specific parts of the body? Who doesn't want to have fun while they tone up their bodies and become healthier in the process? In this chapter, I will outline positions for working out the problem areas you need to focus on.

Position #21. A Quads Workout Position

Your quadriceps are the large muscles in your thighs, and it turns out there's a sex position that's perfect for giving them a good workout. It's similar to the female on top position, but you want to shift it into something more like a frog position. Sure, it doesn't sound like the most attractive looking thing in the world, but it works.

How to do this position: The female gets on top of the male and instead of resting her legs on the bed, she places the soles of her feet flat. As she moves in a bouncing fashion, this position turns into an advanced squat work out. This will mostly focus on the quads.

A variation to try: For extra calorie burning, you can switch your motions from up and down to back and worth. This will work your muscles out even more and contribute to the fat burning of the position.

Position #22. A Chest Workout Position

The greatest opportunity for working out your chest as a man is doing the doggy style position and making a few slight changes. This will tone up your chest area and give you a nice workout.

How to do this position: The woman is on her hands and knees with the man behind her. He can either kneel on the surface or stand by it. This position gives a great chance to work out your upper body since you're using your arms to hold yourself up. Instead of not holding onto anything or placing your hands on your hips, support your weight on your arms and work your chest muscles.

A variation to try: To make this even more of an effective challenge, you can try doing pushups in between. This will work much better on firm beds or other hard surfaces.

Position #23. A Glutes and Hamstrings Position

If you would like to focus on your lower body (specifically your hamstrings and glute muscles), this is a great position for you. This position involves the woman on top and either a chair or a sturdy couch for leverage and support.

How to do this position: To effectively carry out this position, the female should get herself into a lunge position. The man will sit atop whatever surface the couple chooses (a strong chair or nice couch is ideal), and place one foot on the ground and the other on the surface. This will work the glute on one side and the hamstring on the other. Then, you can switch legs so that you're working out each side.

A variation to try: A low-lying couch or chair will provide a great work out, but if you want to make it even more of a challenge and also work your calf muscles, try a high backed chair.

Position #24. A Lower Abs Workout Position

This involves the man sitting cross legged on the floor and also takes a bit of inspiration from a yoga pose called the lotus. If you try this position, you will notice that your lower abdominal muscles get a great work out.

How to do this position: The woman needs to face the man and sit on his lap, straddling him, as he is sitting cross-legged on the floor or a firm surface. Her arms will be wrapped around his body tightly. Focusing on the lower abdominal muscles to power the motion in her pelvis will give her a great workout.

A variation to try: Try switching from up and down to back and forth motions. Each movement creates a different benefit, so play around with options and branch out.

Position #25. Triceps Workout Position

If your arms are the part of your body that needs some work, we have a position for you to try. This is related to the above position that instructs you to work out your lower abs.

How to do this position: Remain in the lotus position with the man cross-legged and the woman wrapped around him, but this time the woman should lean her body backward and have her hands flat on the ground or bed.

A variation to try: Bend your elbows to get the optimum workout from this particular sex position.

Position #26. Hip Flexors Workout Position

For this one, you're engaging in an isometric exercise. What this means is that your muscles are held in a stationary position instead of moving, similar to many yoga positions where benefits are reaped by holding a pose. This position is very effective for strengthening the hip flexor area and needs to be alternated to work out each side of your body equally and receive the best benefits.

How to do this position: For this one, you will want to get into a scissors-like pose, where both parties are lying on their sides. For example, if they man is on his left side and you're lying on your right, you will hold your arm out at a 35 degree angle, instead of resting it on his body.

A variation to try: You can make this workout even more effective by quickly alternating legs. To do this, you will need to get into a groove with your partner, which requires discussion before action.

Position #27. An Upper Abs Workout Position

This one is highly effective, but it's necessary that the person doing it has a good amount of flexibility in their hamstrings. You will want to do a bit of a warm up before attempting this by touching your toes a few times and stretching out your legs in general.

How to do this position: The woman must lie on her back and place the backsides of her upper legs against the man's chest area. She will then want to lift her head and shoulders up into a crunch-like motion. This is a great stomach-toning exercise to do.

A variation to try: She can choose between sticking her feet directly upward into the air or bending them over her partner's backside. This all depends on what is most comfortable to her.

Position #28. A Deltoids Workout Position

This is another position that draws inspiration from the good old fashioned doggy style sex position, only with an added element of excitement. This will tone your shoulders up very quickly if you stick with it and do it frequently.

How to do this position: The woman needs to be on all fours on the couch or bed as the man stands behind her. He will then grab her thighs and lift them up as he pumps back and forth.

Instead of supporting her weight with her entire body, she will only be able to use her upper body, which will strengthen the deltoids.

A variation to try: To make this even more challenging for advanced fitness lovers, the woman can balance herself on her forearms instead of her hands. The man can also intensify the work out by standing without using the couch or bed for support for his legs.

Position #29. A Glutes Workout Position

This one doesn't take any special knowledge, and is quite simple, even for people who may be out of shape. It involves pumping up a classic position into something a bit more advanced.

How to do this position: The woman should lie on her back with her butt in the air, her feet at the edge of the bed, and the man can kneel in front of her, between her legs. He enters her and stays still as she pumps up and down, working out her butt muscles.

A variation to try: To keep it interesting and make sure both parties are getting a workout, you can take turns making the motions.

Position #30. A Position for a Total Body Workout

This is the one you should advance to once you've already got the hang of the basic arch detailed above. Instead of lying flat on your back though, you will be more engaged, creating a thorough and intense work out.

How to do this position: Get into the missionary sex position. The woman should lift her butt off the bed but use her arms to allow her to raise her shoulders and head off the bed, as well. This is similar to a plank workout, but facing the opposite way. Her partner will be supporting himself with his arms while she balances on her limbs.

A variation to try: One way to intensify this workout is to pause every so often and hold your positions, similar to isometric workouts. This will give your muscles an extra challenge and benefit.

Chapter 5

Advanced Sex Positions

For those of you who are ready to take your bed skills up a notch, these are great to try. They are best performed with someone you feel comfortable with. Trying out these fun and exciting positions can be a great way to get closer to someone and deepen your relationship.

Position #31. The Pretzel Twist Position

This is a position which combines elements of familiar positions such as the typical face to face scenario as well as doggy style. This position is great due to its versatility.

How to do this position: The woman should lie on her side as the man kneels and straddles whichever leg of hers is flat on the bed. She will then wrap her other leg around him. This gives the couple much freedom to adjust their movements to whatever feels best.

A variation to try: This position gets even more interesting when you have a mirror next to the bed. Try this out and see how it vamps up your sex life. Feel free to experiment with this versatile position.

Position #32. The Spider

Spiders aren't the first thing that most people would want to associate with sex, but this one is fun, I promise.

How to do this position: Both partners need to be sitting on the bed or couch, facing each other with their legs facing each other. They will lean back on their hands to support their bodies, similar to a crab-walk style stance. Next, the woman will need to move her feet so that they're on either side of the man's hips and also lying flat on the surface you're on.

A variation to try: Instead of thrusting, try rocking back and forth. This will give you the ability to hold eye contact while also seeing what's going on between you. This also gives the female a high level of control over the motions and angle.

Position #33. The Backwards Cross-Legged Adventure

For this position, the man will be seated cross legged on the floor, with the woman on top.

How to do this position: As the guy sits on the floor with his penis facing upward, the woman should turn around so that she is kneeling with her shins against the man's crossed legs. She will lower herself onto him and rock back and forth, using her arms and hands on the floor as support.

A variation to try: This can be done either facing forward or backward and switching back and forth between the two is great fun.

Position #34. The Vixen Position

For this position, you'll need a counter and possibly yoga lessons, but we don't call this section advanced for nothing.

How to do this position: The man needs to be facing the countertop as the woman is sitting on the edge of the ledge. The guy's legs need to be bent slightly and spaced a few feet apart from each other. She will place her arms on his shoulders and his arms will go around her body. She will then prop one of her legs up on his shoulder.

A variation to try: This can be done with either both legs propped upon his shoulders or only one at a time. It all depends on how comfortable and flexible you are.

Position #35. The Stair Master

This position requires that you live somewhere with a staircase or can find one to use. The unique steps and heights offered by this position allow for great G spot penetration.

How to do this position: Both partners should kneel on a staircase with both bodies turned the same way and facing the stairs. The woman can support her body on the stairs in front of her or the banister, as he holds onto her hips for support.

A variation to try: This position offers a great opportunity for the woman to touch her own clitoris. She simply needs to hold onto the banister with one hand and herself with the other.

Position #36. The Inverted Upright Position

For this position, the woman needs to lie flat on her back with her face toward the ceiling. This advanced position involves some interesting upside down movements.

How to do this position: She needs to lie back with her hands supporting her lower back, and lift her legs and butt into the air to be as equal with the ground as possible. He will kneel before her, grab her lower legs and position his knees to be level with her shoulders.

A variation to try: For extra steady leverage and balance, the man can hold onto the woman's hips. She can then hold onto his upper legs and ease of adjustment.

Position #37. X-Rated Position

This position is one you'd never think of trying, but it's great fun once you get the complicated mechanics down.

How to do this position: The man should lie face up on the bed or couch as the woman turns her body around to straddle his body with her back toward him. Now she will lower herself onto his erection and extend her feet backward in the direction of his face and shoulders. Her torso should rest between his feet on the bed. She can now slide back and forth while using his legs to extra leverage and support.

Position #38. Deep Water Fun

This is a fun position to do when you and your partner are swimming together. Chlorinated sources of water may cause infections, so be careful and try to opt for a more natural spot.

How to do this position: Next time you're in water with your partner, find a spot where the water is about chest high on both of you. They will then face each other, with her hands on his shoulders and her legs wrapped around his upper legs or hips. He can now hold onto her rear to keep her steady as he enters her. The weightlessness of the water is great and takes away all strain.

A variation to try: To make this position extra exciting or challenging, you can walk to more shallow water and have her lean her body back as he supports her with his arms.

Position #39. The Propeller Position

This position is a spinoff of the missionary position, but quite a bit more advanced.

How to do this position: The male will climb atop the woman, entering her in the familiar, traditional missionary way. Once he has entered her, he will start spinning his body a full 360 degrees. As he is rotating his body, she will help him with his balance, being sure to lift his legs above her head to prevent injuries. Think of a propeller on a helicopter.

A variation to try: You can mix this position up by having the female be on top and do the same motions. Some couples may find this easier based on their heights and body types.

Position #40. The Slide Position

This position allows for a lot of variations, letting you choose who will be in control and who gets to relax and be surprised.

How to do this position: For the slide position, the female will lie down on the floor (with a blanket beneath her) or the bed on her stomach. Her legs will be straight out from her body and held apart slightly. The guy will then kneel directly behind her butt with his hands to each side of his body, supporting him. Next, he will lean his body backward to join his pelvis with hers. As he thrusts back and forth, you can bring your legs together to fit even tighter together.

A variation to try: She can rest on her elbows, her arms extended in front of her body for extra support and leverage. If the male enjoys dominating, this variation will allow him that freedom. He can slide backward and forward at the speed he chooses, using her thighs as a runway path.

Chapter 6

The Best Sex Positions to Get Pregnant

Everyone knows that getting pregnant when you're "trying" can be difficult and a bit stressful. If you've been giving it a shot you're your partner lately and haven't had any luck, it could be a simple matter of changing your choice of positions. Although it's often overlooked, the positions you have sex in largely determine whether or not you will conceive.

If you are trying to get pregnant, the first and most important rule is to have a lot of sex during your most fertile time period. Chart this out on a calendar based on your cycle so you know which days you are ovulating and should focus on getting busy. Apart from centering your sex life around your fertile days, you should also find positions that allow for the deepest penetration. It's also important that the woman should have an orgasm during sex, since the spasms that come afterward help the sperm reach her egg more effectively.

Position #41. The Magical Mountain Position

Think of the classic doggy style sex position, only with a twist. This pose allows for deep, satisfying penetration, and simultaneous G spot and clitoris attention. Most positions only allow for one or the other, so this arrangement is a pleasure paradise for the woman.

How to do this position: The man will bend over her with his chest pressed up against her back. She will be bent over the bed, possibly with pillows for extra stability under her chest. The pillows allow for her to relax more and relinquish control, but without them she will receive a nice workout.

A variation to try: You can do this both with and without pillows for differing sensations. He can try straightening his body or bending over her for variance, as well. You can also switch up the tempo and pace to keep it interesting, and easily transition into other positions from the magical mountain pose.

Position #42. The Anvil Position

This position will make sure the man is deeply and effectively penetrating the G spot, which is necessary for getting pregnant.

How to do this position: The woman lies on her back as the man climbs atop her. She will then lift her legs into the air, making sure they're up above her head level as the man enters her. He will then hold her ankles together as he holds her joined legs to one side. This creates a very tight sensation for him.

Position #43. The Spooning Position

This is another basic and well known position with wonderful benefits for strengthening intimacy and getting pregnant.

How to do this position: The man should be positioned behind her as she is lying down which will help the chances of his sperm reaching her egg. It's like the typical spooning position but tilted forward a bit. After he has ejaculated, she should roll onto her back to help the sperm travel to the egg.

A variation to try: For variance, the couple can try having her spread her legs wider, or even having him flip onto his back so that she is on top of him while facing up.

Position #44. The Butterfly Position for Contraception

This position involves a table and two partners hoping to conceive a child. It follows the guidelines of gravity, as far as ideals for sperm reaching the cervix area.

How to do this position: She will lie back on a table in the house as the guy gets in between her legs. He will then raise her pelvis using his hands (or he could place pillows under her, instead).

A variation to try: An added element that could make this position more effective is the female holding her position for a while after the man ejaculates inside of her. This will make the success of the sperm reaching the egg more likely.

Position #45. The Plough Position

This position is best if you are fit and flexible, but it can be achieved with some practice with your partner. It's also necessary that you trust them to hold you up!

How to do this position: The female will need to stand on her hands with her legs in the air. Having something to lean against might be helpful, at first. The man will get in between her legs and enter her from there, supporting her hips with his hands.

A variation to try: This can be done in the middle of the room or against a surface, depending on how flexible and strong each partner is. The effect of gravity makes it a conception-friendly position.

Position #46. The Headboard Mambo

This position involves the women's feet up against the wall and the man kneeling in front of her. It's a great position to try for aspiring parents. Not only is it good for chances of conceiving, but it works out the woman's legs quite well.

How to do this position: The woman needs to lie down on her back against the bed, with her feet facing the wall and headboard of the bed. She should raise her pelvis off of this surface

A variation to try: To aid the insemination, you can place some pillows under your lower back and stay still for a while after sex so that the sperm cannot flow downward out of you.

Position #47. The Wheelbarrow

It's been said that the man being on top increasing the likelihood of pregnancy. This is due to the belief that these positions allow for the man to deeply penetrate and for the sperm to get as close to the cervix as possible. This means that the sperm will have a head start on their journey toward the egg. This is why the wheelbarrow is great for partners hoping to become parents.

How to do this position: The wheelbarrow position involves the woman on the ground in a arrangement similar to a push up. The man will grab her ankles and press their pelvises together, entering her from behind as he pumps in and out. Since, again, this is a position where gravity is working with the sperm's journey, it will be beneficial for conception.

A variation to try: This is easiest to do on the floor, but for couples with advanced stamina, it's possible for the woman to be leaning her arms on a bed instead. Depending on the height of the partners involved, this could be a more harmonious arrangement.

Position #48. Downward Dog

This is another twist on a famous yoga position. The woman's feet are flat on the floor and so are her hands. This yoga position allows for every major muscle group in the body to be stretched out, but it can also be an effective position for getting pregnant since the woman's head is lower than her uterus and the sperm will naturally flow downward. The woman has to have some what strong arms for this position to be comfortable.

How to do this position: As the woman is in the downward dog yoga position with her feet face down, palms down, and butt in the air (so that her body makes an upside down V shape), the man can get behind her. She needs to make sure her legs are spread adequately for him to fit between them. He can hold her hips to help her stay balanced since the motion might compromise sturdiness.

A variation to try: The man can get some good stretching in and join in the yoga fun by lifting his arms and holding them there. The tautness of holding this stance while simultaneously thrusting will work out his abs along with his legs. If she feels as though her arms are receiving too much pressure, it's possible to hold onto a low=lying surface.

Position #49. The Standing Pleasure Embrace

This may be difficult for some couples depending on their level of fitness and stamina. It also works best if the man weighs more than the woman and is a bit taller than her. It can work if they are equal heights as long as he is heavier.

How to do this position: The man stands up and the woman is behind held by him with her legs wrapped around him. He enters her and uses the strength of his legs to power his thrusts. This is very intimate because she is being completely supported by him. The position allows for deep penetration which is of utmost importance in attempting to conceive a baby.

A variation to try: If the man finds that his arms are getting tired or sore from supporting her entire body weight, he can lean backwards against a wall or other hip-high surface. She can also place her arms against the wall to take a bit of her weight off him.

Position #50. Classic Doggy

We saved this one for the end, because although it's well known, it's one of the best in terms of pleasure for both partners, stamina, and also getting pregnant.

How to do this position: The classic doggy is quite self-explanatory, and means the woman is on her knees bent forward and the man enters from behind.

A variation to try: The importance in turning this into a baby-making position is making sure you're in the right positions for optimal effect. If the male ejaculates inside of the woman with her back half at a higher angle than her head, the sperm travels downward toward the egg.

Conclusion

Thank you again for purchasing this wonderful and informative book!

I hope this book was able to help you to get some new ideas for spicing up your sex life and impressing your partner. Sex is an extremely important aspect of any adult relationship, and couples with more active intimacy are happier in general. Great sex is good for your body, mind, spirit, and relationship. In the modern times of high divorce rates, it can be easy to get discouraged about maintaining a satisfying sex life and thus a happy partnership. Who doesn't want to have a long, healthy marriage? Although the statistics look grim, and many people lose interest in sex with their long term partners over time, this scenario does not have to apply to you.

With the knowledge I will give you in this book, you don't have to settle for anything less than amazing when it comes to sex with your partner. Keeping sex lives interesting takes effort. For this reason, it's best to stay creative and open to new things when it comes to sex. It can be hard to know exactly what to do, so guidebooks such as this are necessary sometimes. Sometimes, it only takes the right spark to get the fire going.

The next step is to take what you've learned in this book and apply it to your life. With these specific instructions, you should be well on your way to stepping up your game in the bedroom. All it takes is a willing, adventurous partner, some new information, and you're on your way to a fulfilled and exciting sex life.

Finally, if you enjoyed this book, please take the time to share your thoughts and post a review on Amazon. You can take this opportunity to speak the knowledge you've gained and help others. It'd be greatly appreciated!

Thank you and good luck!

www.ingramcontent.com/pod-product-compliance
Lightning Source LLC
Chambersburg PA
CBHW071113280526
45787CB00003B/1013